JUST EAT IT

How to Ditch the Green Smoothies & Juice Fasts, Heal Your Gut and Enjoy Eating Again

By Joey Lott

www.joeylotthealth.com

2

Publishing services provided by 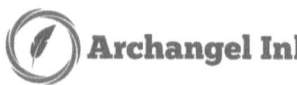 Archangel Ink

ISBN: 1518665985
ISBN-13: 978-1518665981

Table of Contents

4

Getting Out of Digestive Hell

Digestive hell sucks. If you've ever visited, then you know what I mean. Through the various stages of digestive hell, I experienced bloating, heaviness, extreme flatulence, constipation, painful diarrhea, heartburn, vomiting, nausea, stagnation, mucus, burning, jabbing pain, and more. I went from being a kid who could eat half a chicken, a plateful of mashed potatoes, and a few slices of cake all in one sitting to struggling to eat even 1500 calories a day after more than a decade of dietary hijinks. I felt terrible most of the time, and I became obsessed with trying to fix my digestive problems. I thought about food all the time, but I couldn't figure out how to eat it without feeling terrible.

Digestive hell is littered with billboards and commercials advertising for things that promise a one-way ticket to digestive paradise. I tried them. Most didn't help at all. In fact, most made things worse. A few of them seemed to help for a while, but then I found myself deposited into another corner of digestive hell, back to square one or worse. The things I tried included supplemental digestive enzymes, more fiber, fiber supplements, herbal "cleanses," fasting, juicing, veganism, raw milk diet, raw food, paleo, GAPS, low carb, whole food, no sugar, no salt, yoga, weight lifting, "digestive" spices, colonics (yikes!), apple cider vinegar, lemon juice, herbal bitters, and more.

Does any of this sound familiar to you? Are you tired of feeling terrible, always thinking about food but terrified of eating it because of the way you feel when you do? Do you worry find yourself reading lots of websites about candida cleanses or Ayurvedic lifestyle cures or spiritual healing in hopes that something, *anything*, might help you to feel good again? Heck, maybe you'd settle for just *decent* or even plain old *not bad*!

What I'll share with you in this book is how I finally found my way to digestive wellness without expensive supplements, cultish diets, or ultra restrictions. No juicers were necessary. No rebounders. No enemas or anything else going into the rectum. No spinning classes. No hot yoga. No need to make bone broth day in and day out. No fasting. Nothing particularly unpleasant at all.

Here's what I found: The primary factors in digestive health are low metabolic rate and stress. When I say "stress," I am referring to the physiological experience of hormonal changes that take place under a variety of circumstances. Some of the major contributors to stress are poor psychological adaptation, lack of sleep, chronic hyperventilation, allergic or "autoimmune" reactions, over-exercise, chronic physical tension, and *not eating enough*.

In this book, I'll share with you some of the main ways I found to restore digestive health. I've done a great deal of research, reading through lots of clinical human trials, and much of what I share with you in this book is grounded in hypotheses that have borne out real-world testing in humans. I have also talked with a *lot* of people who have digestive problems--many much worse than I ever experienced--and the suggestions that I give you in this book are the things that have helped a lot of the people I speak with feel much better.

With all that said, I'm not promising you a miracle cure. What is required is some honesty and honest evaluation of your present choices and lifestyle. If you already eat 3000 or more calories a day of a variety of real foods (including fat, protein, and carbohydrates), you are eating an omnivorous diet, you sleep 8 or more hours a night, you don't worry or get anxious about things, you don't exercise for more than 30 minutes every other day, and your temperature is consistently 98.6 F (37 C) or above while your resting pulse is 75-85, then the advice in this book probably won't help you. Or, if you currently restrict your diet (vegan, low carb, GAPS, etc.) and are unwilling to be more inclusive, then this book cannot help you. Or, if you insist on depriving yourself of sleep or running for an hour a day, then this book cannot help you. In other words, you have to be willing to admit that what you are doing isn't working and be willing to make some changes.

By and large, the changes that I will suggest are *pleasant* changes. I'm going to recommend that you eat more, rest more, relax more, laugh more, and let your belly hang out instead of sucking it in all the time. Along with these changes, I'm going to explain why many of the things you've tried or thought about trying generally won't work. So I'll be debunking a lot of the stuff that gets touted as the cures for digestive problems. My hope is that you'll see that healthy digestion begins with an enjoyable, sustainable lifestyle that includes enough food and rest and enjoyment so that you'll stop torturing yourself with all the stuff you think that you're supposed to do in order to be healthy.

Finally, before we get started, I want to mention that this book is specifically for people who experience "mysterious" digestive problems like I used to. In these cases, I'm fairly confident that what follows will likely be helpful to you. On the other hand, this book is *not* specifically designed for those with Crohn's disease, celiac disease, or other inflammatory bowel disorders. The advice that I give in this book will undoubtedly be helpful for people with those conditions since reductions in stress and inflammation and improvements in metabolic health are likely to help just about anyone. However, since I don't have first-hand experience with those conditions, I am unable to give recommendations specific to those conditions.

I also won't cover remedies in this book for specific types of infections that can affect digestion. For example, I don't go into detail on what to do about helicobacter pylori infections because this is not a medical book. Instead, this is a book that describes simple, non-restrictive things that you can do that will improve metabolic rate, reduce stress, and improve digestion for most people. And, as it turns out, these things will likely improve immune function and reduce inflammation, which *may* help with any infections that may be present.

Metabolic Downregulation

During World War II, some researchers at the University of Minnesota conducted a landmark study with healthy human volunteers. For six months, the volunteers (all young men) were fed a diet of 1600 calories a day. The results were startling. Although the goal was to drastically reduce the men's weight, everyone was surprised to find that the men exhibited all the physiological and psychological signs of starvation. Among the many changes noted was that the men had an average reduction in basal metabolic rate of 40 percent! Although the volunteers were striving to reduce their weight by 25 percent, they were unable to achieve their goal because drastically reduced metabolic rates stalled their weight loss beyond a certain point.

Basal metabolic rate (or BMR) refers to the rate at which energy is created and utilized by the body. The BMR determines how much energy must be consumed in order to maintain basic bodily functions, including respiration, heartbeat, and keeping the brain alive. When the BMR is low, fewer calories are used. Of course, in times of famine or starvation, having a low BMR is highly advantageous because it keeps the body alive even when food is scarce. This way, the body lives another day in hopes that food will become available soon.

But unfortunately, low BMR comes with a lot of unpleasant symptoms as well, including those exhibited by the starving Minnesotans such as increased hypochondria, food obsession, anxiety, aggression, heat and cold intolerance, insomnia, falling hair, fatigue, frequent urination, aches and pains, and more.

At the other end of the spectrum a researcher named Ethan Sims conducted experiments in the state prison system in Vermont beginning in the 1960s that mirrored the starvation experiments in Minnesota. But instead of starving volunteers, Sims asked for volunteers who wanted to eat as much as they could for months on end. During this experiment, volunteers ate as much as 10,000 calories a day with the goal of gaining 25 percent of their starting weight. But much as the Minnesotans were unable to lose 25 percent of their weight, the Vermonters were unable to gain 25 percent of their weight. The Vermonters' BMRs *increased* by 50 percent!

With dramatically increased metabolisms, the Vermonters were able to eat *massive* amounts of food without gaining weight. In fact, after their metabolisms were revved up, they had to continue to eat 8,000 to 10,000 calories a day *just to maintain* their increased weights.

These same findings have been duplicated a number of times since these experiments, including some important experiments conducted by Rudolph Leibel, a medical doctor and researcher and the discoverer of leptin, the so-called "satiety hormone." While at Rockefeller University, Leibel conducted an experiment in which he was able to closely monitor the BMR of various volunteers, and what he found was that BMRs change according to various factors, including how much a person eats.

One of the things to note is that lowered BMRs generally *decrease* digestive function whereas raised BMRs *increase* digestive function. Many people who struggle with digestive problems have low BMRs.

Although there are a number of ways to measure basal metabolic rate, the easiest way to measure your own metabolic rate is to track your basal temperature and your resting pulse rate. If either is low, it is a good indicator of low BMR. You can track your basal temperature by taking your oral temperature first thing in the morning *before getting out of bed* and after having slept without artificial heating elements such as an electric blanket or a waterbed. If your basal temperature is consistently below 97.8 F (36.6 C), then you have a low BMR.

You can track resting pulse by placing your index and middle fingers on any of the major arteries and counting the beats per minute. The best arteries are the radial artery on the wrist or the carotid arteries on the side of the throat. If your resting pulse is under 75, that may signify a low BMR. If your pulse is higher than 85, that may also indicate a low BMR because a raised pulse rate can be caused by stress hormones that are common with a low BMR.

If *either* the temperature or the pulse is low, that is a very good indicator of low BMR. As we've just seen, one common way in which to lower BMR is through under-eating, which is what we'll explore in the next section.

Eating More

Paradoxically, one way to improve digestion is to *eat more*. Although it is certainly possible to have digestive problems while eating 4000 calories a day (particularly if lots of those calories are from industrially-produced food such as high fructose corn syrup or omega-6 polyunsaturated "vegetable" oils such as canola, corn, or soy), it's far *more* likely that people experiencing major digestive problems are not eating enough.

In this day and age with plentiful food and with warnings right and left that we should be *reducing* our food intake, it may seem strange to suggest that people eat more. However, the fact is that the majority of people I communicate with who are experiencing digestive problems are eating less than they need to to fuel a healthy metabolic rate.

How much food is enough? This is a difficult question to answer with a one-size-fits-all response because it seems that some people in some places are able to eat less and remain healthy while others need more. For example, a group of people on a Pacific island called Kitava were studied because they have no cardiovascular disease or other so-called "diseases of civilization." The researchers catalogued everything about the Kitavans' lifestyle and dietary habits, and among the things that they found, they reported that the men were eating an average of 2500 calories per day while the women were eating slightly less.

On the other hand, when we look at the Minnesota Starvation Experiment, the researchers found that during the pre-starvation phase of the experiment the men had to eat 3200 calories per day in order to maintain a healthy weight. And in the Vermont studies, the researchers reported that prior to overfeeding, the men had to eat 3000-4000 calories per day to maintain their weights.

Another experiment that sheds some light on the matter is an experiment in Biosphere, which is an enclosed structure in Arizona that is intended to be entirely self-sufficient. While participants were in the structure for a year, a miscalculation meant that they were unable to produce as much food as they had anticipated. As a result, the participants each ate 2000 calories per day. One of the measurements taken revealed that during their stay in Biosphere, the participants all had a decline in serum T3, which is a hormone that is closely linked with metabolic health. Low levels of T3 are often indicative of starvation. So while there were lots of other factors to take into account, it is possible that the low-calorie diet that the volunteers were eating contributed to low T3 levels. In other words, they needed to eat more to maintain a healthy metabolism.

From all of this, we may start to see a picture start to form. Thus far we haven't come across examples of healthy people who eat less than 2500 calories per day in the long run. Of course, that doesn't mean that it isn't possible to do so. But it does cast some suspicion on any diets that are less than 2500 calories per day in which the person is also experiencing poor health, including digestive problems.

The evidence that I have found in my research suggests that anyone living in a Western culture typically needs substantially more calories than we think. Most men will require 3000 to 4000 calories per day to maintain a healthy metabolic rate. Most women will need between 2500 and 3500 calories per day. Pregnant and nursing mothers will need more than others. And people recovering from illness or people with poor digestion need more than those who are healthy.

The starving Minnesotans needed more than 4000 calories per day (sometimes as much as 11,000 calories in a day) for nine months before they restored their original metabolic rate, weight, and health.

According to these guidelines, do you eat enough? Do you have a history of restricting calories for weight loss (or any other reason)? Have you undergone extended fasts? Have you ever gone through phases of over-exercising (more than 30 minutes every other day) without massive amounts of calories and massive sleep? Have you ever had an extended illness?

If you answered yes to any of the preceding questions, then it is entirely possible that you may need to eat *even more* than 3500-4000 calories per day in order to restore digestive health.

How to Eat More

You may see the potential value in eating more to heal poor digestion, but then you find yourself in a bit of a Catch-22 situation; you need to eat more to improve your digestion, but due to poor digestion, you feel that you cannot eat more! As frustrating as it can be, know that you are not alone, and many people in terrible digestive shape have found ways to eat more and improve their digestion.

In the sections that follow, we'll explore some of the specific things that people do that sabotage their digestion and their ability to eat more. But before we get into those details, let's cover the basics first.

If you are presently eating less than 3500 or 4000 calories a day, then chances are that you're not eating the right things nor enough of the right things. Although we hear a lot about what the right things are--"healthy" whole grains, lots of green vegetables, etc.--in the context of healing digestive function, most of those foods are usually the *wrong* foods to be eating a lot of.

In order to eat more, you have to focus on foods that offer the following qualities: highly palatable, low to moderate fiber, and calorie dense. If you think about it for a second, you'll notice that most kids have no problem eating a *ton* of ice cream, cookies, and candy. How can they do that? Well, for one thing, they have healthy metabolisms. But for another thing, those foods meet all the criteria I just mentioned. Contrast that with kale and brown rice, and you'll see that if your goal is to pack in the calories, ice cream, cookies, and candy win *hands down*.

For a lot of people with digestive problems, it is hard to let go of the idea that they should only be eating "healthy" foods. But as we'll see in the following sections, the insistence of only eating "healthy" foods ends up harming people with compromised metabolisms.

Although ice cream, cookies, and candy are wonderful for packing in calories, I am *not* suggesting that it is necessarily a good idea to eat *only* those things either. Obviously, we need some *balanced* nutrition that includes adequate quality protein, fat, and carbohydrates along with a full complement of vitamins and minerals and other nutrients. But as Ancel Keys, the lead researcher in the Minnesota Starvation Experiment, said, "The character of the rehabilitation diet is important also, but *unless calories are abundant*, then extra proteins, vitamins, and minerals are of little value." In other words, you can eat kale until you're blue in the face and your belly is distended, but you won't get nearly enough calories to heal your body.

In the context of a diet designed to heal the metabolism and digestive system, calories are king. Balanced nutrition is a distant second. This is counter to what we are normally told, but it seems to be true nonetheless.

In the next sections we'll explore some of the specific ways in which people sabotage their digestion, why it doesn't work, and what to do instead. We'll also see the objections that many people have to eating enough calories and why it is important to let go of those objections for the duration of the rehabilitation diet.

Whole Food / Fiber

A *lot* of people are sold on the notion that the only healthy diet is a whole food diet jam-packed with lots of dietary fiber. And, along with that, a lot of people actually take *supplementary* fiber in the form of things such as bran or psyllium husks. This is *completely* counterproductive to any efforts to heal digestion.

While the various types of carbohydrates that occur in fruits and vegetables (including some of the indigestible ones called "fiber") can be good for health in a variety of ways, that doesn't mean that *all* of them are always good. Nor does it mean that more is always better.

One of the problems with dietary fiber from a rehabilitative diet perspective is that it is indigestible, which means that your body cannot extract energy from it. Think about it for a second; you wouldn't be able to survive for long if all you ate was tree bark because you cannot extract energy from it. So even if small amounts of *some types* of fiber may be helpful at times, *too much* simply fills you up without giving you the thing you *most* need, which is calories.

The second problem with some types of fiber, particularly bulking fibers such as bran (i.e. whole grains) or psyllium husks, is that they can actually worsen digestion over time. These types of fiber are popular because they can *initially* reduce transit time and increase fecal mass. Pooping often and massively has become synonymous with health for many people, and so the initial effects of bulking fiber can seem desirable.

Unfortunately, the way in which bulking fiber causes these effects is by *stretching and irritating* the digestive system. So over time, increasing amounts of bulking fiber are needed to produce the same effects. And, eventually, all the irritation and stretching can actually reduce the natural function of the digestive system. John Harvey Kellogg was the co-inventor of corn flakes and a medical doctor who ran a health resort in Battle Creek, Michigan in which he promoted the fanatical adherence to diets composed of large amounts of dietary fiber. Over time, he discovered that the diet actually *produced* constipation rather than curing it, and so he remedied that problem by adding *mineral oil* to the diets. (Mineral oil is a petroleum by-product that, when ingested, inhibits absorption of nutrients. So I don't recommend trying Kellogg's approach.)

As we'll see shortly, *some* types of indigestible carbohydrates are a valuable part of a diet *in moderation*. However, there are some types of fiber that simply don't seem to offer much value to most people, and during a rehabilitative diet, it is generally best to minimize or eliminate these types of fiber. Bran from whole grains, psyllium husk, flax seed, and other substances marketed as bulking fiber are the worst offenders.

During a rehabilitative diet, it is generally best to focus on low to moderate fiber foods or foods that contain no dietary fiber along with some whole fruits and vegetables that will provide all the indigestible carbohydrates that are needed. Meat, butter, cheese, cream, fruit juice, sugar, and white rice are all examples of foods that contain substantial amounts of energy (calories) with minimal dietary fiber. And, as we'll see, all of these foods have the added benefit of being real foods rather than industrial food products.

Low-Carb

I don't need to tell you that low-carb is a trend that keeps on trending. From Atkins to South Beach to variations on the paleo trend, *lots* of people are promoting the low carb agenda. They present their pitches in such a way that many of us have become convinced that carbohydrates cause everything from fatness to cancer to Alzheimer's.

In the short term, low-carb diets can sometimes produce impressive results. People can drop pounds, gain muscle, have loads of energy, and on and on. But over time, low-carb diets typically lead to crashes for most people. That's because for *most* of us, our ancestors evolved over tens of thousands of years eating carbohydrates. Even in high latitude conditions, our ancestors ate what carbohydrates they could during the warm months.

Some of us may be able to go for a month or two or six eating very low-carb. But sooner or later, the honeymoon phase wears off and we're left with the aftermath. During low-carb diets, some people, particularly if they have a lot of adipose (fat) tissue, may enter a ketogenic state that can produce many of the beneficial effects attributed to low-carb diets. However, once the fat stores run low or if fatty acid respiration is impaired, things don't feel so good.

What's more, I've come across a few clinical human trials that compare the effects of low-fat diets versus low-carbohydrate diets versus low-nothing diets, and what they typically report is that stress hormone levels rise considerably during low-carbohydrate diets. Over time, that results in worsening health, including impaired digestion.

There's another reason why insufficient carbohydrates can cause problems, specifically digestive problems. Over millions of years, humans evolved alongside other life forms. We developed mutually beneficial relationships with many of them. And it turns out that *90 percent* of the cells in the human body *aren't human!* Nine tenths of the cells in our bodies are bacteria without which we cannot survive. And a large number of those bacteria live in the digestive system. In fact, the average adult human's large intestine is lined with nearly *four pounds* of bacteria that we need in order to survive.

The bacteria in our intestines is made up of an amazing variety of species--*way* more than those probiotic products contain. These bacteria need food to survive. And what the bacteria eat is *fermentable, indigestible* carbohydrates. In other words, they actually eat some types of fiber and other resistant carbohydrates.

What that means is that if you don't eat enough carbohydrates, a good portion of the 90 percent of the cells that make up your body will start to die. And since those cells are an important part of your immune system and the manner in which you digest and eliminate, you need carbs.

The bacteria don't like bran and psyllium because they can't eat things like that. What they like are the types of carbohydrates found in fruits, vegetables, and starches.

Now, of course, that doesn't mean you should be pounding down apples and kale just because your friendly bacteria are hungry. A little goes a long way. But neither should you eliminate nor greatly reduce your dietary carbohydrates just because you read a book that says that your caveman ancestors only ate wooly mammoth hearts.

In general, people who want to improve digestion will do well to eat more of *everything*, including carbohydrates. That includes easily digested carbohydrates like sugar and fruit juice as well as starches and whole fruits to provide food for intestinal bacteria.

Veganism and Protein

Veganism is another way that many people sabotage their digestion. Among the ways that veganism can harm digestion are insufficient fat-soluble vitamins (especially pre-formed vitamin A and vitamin K2), insufficient dietary cholesterol, and insufficient quality protein. As a former long-term, committed vegan, I am very aware of how unwelcomed these arguments are. However, I also assure you that these problems can contribute to real digestive problems.

Vitamin A is needed for health across the board. Although it is theoretically possible to convert carotenoids (e.g. beta-carotene) from plants into true vitamin A (retinol), many people, *especially* vegans, are poor converters. Therefore, the only truly reliable sources of vitamin A are animal foods. One of the best sources is liver. In fact, it is so concentrated that it is not advisable to eat too much liver too often. Generally, four ounces of liver every week or two is sufficient. Other decent sources include butter and egg yolks as well as whole milk. Including these foods in your diet can help ensure that you are getting true vitamin A.

Vitamin K2 is only found in animal foods (or some foods fermented by bacteria, such as natto). Although humans can theoretically convert vitamin K1, found in vegetables, into K2, there is reason to suspect that the conversion is generally insufficient to meet needs. Therefore, including animal foods in one's diet is the only way to ensure adequate vitamin K2 (unless one wants to eat natto, that is).

Dietary cholesterol has been much maligned in recent decades, but now it is being exonerated by researchers. Dietary cholesterol does not significantly alter plasma (blood) cholesterol levels. Instead, dietary cholesterol provides the body with a substance that is needed for *every cell in the body*. Cholesterol is used to form cellular membranes to shield nerves, to build natural hormones in the body such as testosterone, and *to digest food*. The liver secretes a substance called bile, which is essential for the body to be able to absorb dietary fats and nutrients. In fact, bile is so precious that the body reabsorbs approximately 95 percent of what the liver secretes so that it can be used again. And bile is made of cholesterol.

The only dietary sources of cholesterol are animal foods. Among the best sources of cholesterol are egg yolks and liver.

Along with cholesterol, another important nutrient is choline. Choline is needed for a large number of functions in the body, including numerous digestive functions. Choline is important for supporting metabolic balance, including insulin sensitivity. And choline is needed in large amounts by the liver. Choline deficiencies are linked with non-alcoholic fatty liver disease.

Although there are some plant sources of choline, the only truly abundant dietary sources of the nutrient are animal foods. Specifically, egg yolks and liver (as well as other organs such as kidneys) are superior sources of choline.

Finally, let's look at the protein issue. Sufficient *quality* dietary protein is essential for digestive health. The *only* thing that increases stomach acid production is protein, and as we'll see later, insufficient stomach acid production has a whole host of problems that come along with it. Insufficient protein means insufficient stomach acid. Dietary protein also prevents the body from breaking down muscle to meet its protein requirements. If you don't eat enough dietary protein, then you tax your body's capacities.

Quality protein is protein with a complete and balanced amino acid profile. While it is *theoretically* possible to obtain sufficient complete protein on a vegan diet, in practice it simply doesn't happen no matter how much beans and rice one eats. Let's put this in perspective; to avoid protein deficiency, a person needs about 0.8 grams of protein per kilogram of body mass. That means that an 80 kilogram (175 pound) person needs to eat 64 grams of complete protein each day just to avoid protein deficiency. That's a minimum. More is preferable, particularly for anyone who is recovering from poor digestion.

One *cup* of dried pinto beans gives about 40 grams of protein. That's incomplete protein, though. So to complete the missing amino acids you'll need to add a cup of rice. Once you cook the beans, that's *three* cups of cooked beans. And once you cook the rice that's *two* cups of cooked rice. You'll need to eat all of that just to get approximately 40 grams of protein. That's *a lot* of beans and rice, and you'll still be less than two thirds of the way to your *minimum* protein requirements for the day.

Now, compare that to a third pound hamburger with a slice of cheddar and a few slices of bacon. That contains approximately the same amount of protein, but in a *much* easier to eat form. It wouldn't be terribly challenging for most people to figure out how to eat two of those in a day, which would yield enough protein to not only avoid protein deficiency, but also provide some protein to *rebuild* the digestive system.

Although there isn't a great deal of talk of protein deficiency in places such as North America, that's mostly because the majority of the population eats *a tremendous* amount of protein. But there is an increasing number of people who are protein deficient and don't even know it. Keep track of what you eat, and add up the *complete* protein in a day. If you are averaging less than 0.8 grams per kilogram of body mass, then you are deficient. Ideally, you should aim for at least 1 gram per kilogram or a bit more.

Now, with all of that said, I know that some committed vegans with digestive problems will read this book and be unwilling to compromise on their principles. First of all, I will encourage you to read my book, *Vegan Recovery*, for a more comprehensive and detailed discussion of the subject, which may give you some peace of mind when it comes to including some animal foods in your diet. You needn't even eat meat if you don't want to since the inclusion of dairy and eggs will help tremendously. But if you still refuse to eat animal foods, then I will make a few suggestions for how to at least minimize the potential negative impacts of a strict vegan diet.

In order to improve your fat-soluble vitamin profile, you're going to want to make sure to *always* eat green and orange vegetables with generous helpings of *saturated* fat sources such as coconut oil or palm oil. That will help to ensure that you maximize your conversion and absorption of the fat-soluble carotenoids and K1 that those vegetables contain. You can also supplement with vegan sources of K2 that are derived from bacterial fermentation, often fermentation of soy. I know of no *natural* vegan source of preformed vitamin A.

Unfortunately, there are *no* vegan sources of cholesterol. And the vegan sources of choline are fairly insignificant with things like beans and broccoli topping the list despite their relatively low levels of the nutrient. So when it comes to choline, you might consider a supplement.

For protein, one of the best quality vegan protein sources is the white potato. Unfortunately, you'd have to eat *a lot* of potatoes to meet your protein needs. But adding some potatoes to your diet will be helpful. White potatoes in place of rice, for example, will yield a similar amount of calories and volume but considerably more nutrition. Otherwise, you'll need to eat *a lot* of beans with rice or potatoes. You can also consider supplementing with a vegan protein powder. Generally, I don't see much to recommend about such things, but if the alternative is to suffer poor health (including digestive problems), then a protein supplement is preferable.

Food Combining

The food combining idea has been around in popular culture for at least a century, and it received a major boost in popularity since the 1970s and 80s with the publication of the book, *Fit for Life*. The notion is that different types of food digest differently and at different rates; therefore, proponents of the theory recommend that one should eat only one type of food at a time, leaving sufficient time for digestion between each meal. For example, advocates will recommend eating nothing but fruit in the morning. They suggest that one should *never* eat protein and carbohydrates together. And they also suggest that dairy should never be combined with anything else. Depending on who is making the recommendations, the rules are more or less strict.

Many people with poor digestion either have tried food combining practices in the past (which usually worsens digestion) or they eventually learn about the idea, hoping that it will provide a solution to the problem.

In the short term, food combining practices *can* seem to offer some relief, particularly if a person has been in the habit of eating insufficient quality protein or if one has low stomach acid for any other reason. In these cases, eating fruit only, for example, can give some relief from the usual bloating and discomfort that can come with a mixed meal for those with weak digestion.

However, the typical practices of food combining (or, rather, *not* combining) generally worsen symptoms over time. The reason is typically two-fold. For one, these practices usually *decrease* the amount of energy (calories) that a person can comfortably eat in a day. Consider that a large breakfast of fruit might only amount to little more than 400 or 500 calories. Due to the high water content, it can be difficult to eat more than that. Or, if one opts for *dried* fruit in order to eat more calories, the nature of that much dried fruit typically leads to digestive discomfort for most people. So the practice will normally cause a decrease in calories, which will further lower BMR, worsening digestion.

The other problem is that food combining practices typically mean that the amount of protein in most meals will be very low. For example, an all-fruit meal will contain negligible protein. And *total* daily protein will also usually drop considerably. A reduction in dietary protein causes metabolic disturbances that are unfavorable. But also, it will lead to a *decrease* in stomach acid production. The result, over time, will be a worsening ability to digest anything other than fruit or fat.

The food combining theory is a seductive one if you aren't familiar with the workings of the digestive tract. However, when you learn about how digestion really works, you may begin to discover that we are *designed* to be able to eat mixed meals. When stomach acid production is adequate, the acid levels break down protein in the stomach while *preventing* any fermentation of carbohydrates. This means that *no* bloating can happen when stomach acid levels are sufficient.

Mixed meals containing protein, carbohydrates, and fat together are generally the *best* way to eat. For one thing, they are more palatable, which means that you'll be able to eat more calories than you would otherwise, and as we've already seen, that's important. For another thing, the combination helps to ensure that everything gets digested and absorbed well. Fats are necessary for the absorption of many nutrients, for example, so if you were to eat fruit or vegetables alone without some good fats, you wouldn't be able to extract the nutrition. Also, many people simply find that eating too much fat or protein without adequate amounts of the other and carbohydrates will leave them feeling nauseous whereas a mixed meal will be just fine. For example, try eating half a stick of butter without anything else. It won't feel very good to most people. But add to that a baked potato to soak up some of the butter and some chicken and onions fried in the butter, and that's much more palatable. In fact, most people could sneak in a tad bit *more* butter that way. So I advise eating mixed meals in order to improve digestion.

Stomach Acid

As we started to see in the previous section, low stomach acid production can be a problem. If stomach acid production is low, then you'll have a hard time digesting protein well, you'll get bloating from eating mixed meals with carbohydrates, you'll be susceptible to bacterial infections from your food, and you may also be susceptible to acid reflux. So improving stomach acid production can help a lot.

The internet and books are full of advice suggesting to use various supplements in order to increase stomach acid. The most popular of these suggestions are apple cider vinegar, lemon juice, and betaine HCl. Of these, there is little reason to suspect that the first two will do much good. The pH of the stomach must drop below 3 before it is acidic enough for protein digestion to happen. Since apple cider vinegar pH is not low enough, it is very unlikely that you could lower your stomach pH sufficiently no matter *how* much of the stuff you drink. Lemon juice, on the other hand, does have a low enough pH. However, after it is diluted by stomach contents, it is unlikely to sufficiently lower stomach pH.

Supplemental betaine HCl contains, as the name states, hydrochloric acid, which is the type of acid the stomach naturally produces. As such, it is tempting to believe that it can lower stomach pH sufficiently. However, it is important to note that HCl is used in a *lot* of supplements and drugs, some of which are designed to *raise* pH, not lower it. So the mere presence of HCl in a supplement does *not* mean it will lower stomach pH.

I have only found *one* human study testing the effects of supplemental betaine HCl on stomach pH. In that one test, supplementing with betaine HCl lowered stomach pH and kept it below 3 for over an hour. The study used only one type of betaine HCl supplement-- one manufactured by Designs for Health. It is unclear, however, whether the effects were due to betaine HCl or not. So until there is further evidence, it is too soon to say whether supplemental betaine HCl will really improve stomach acid levels or not, but it is the most promising option to date.

With all that said, supplements are probably *not* the best way to improve stomach acid production. The things that harm stomach acid production are protein deficiency, insufficient calories, stress, insufficient salt, and insufficient sleep. So these are the things that I would recommend addressing. We'll look more at the stress and sleep components later in the book, and we've already looked at the importance of calories and protein. So here let's examine the salt connection a little more.

Salt provides essential nutrients for digestive health and for the production of hydrochloric acid. When salt intake is insufficient, stomach acid production can suffer. Many people these days restrict salt for a variety of reasons, but for *most* people, salt restriction is completely unnecessary. In fact, for *most* people, salt hasn't actually been shown to adversely affect blood pressure, contrary to popular opinion.

Sodium is one of the major components of salt, and insufficient sodium even has its very own medical term--hyponatremia (Latin for too little sodium). Hyponatremia causes swelling within cells, which can lead to plenty of unpleasantness. The condition can be severe and life-threatening, but in most cases it's mild and might contribute to mild lack of appetite, nausea, or mucus buildup. If you crave salt in the least, it's a good sign that you could do with some more sodium, and salt is a simple, natural, and tasty way to remedy that deficiency.

For some people, adding sufficient salt to food can make a *world* of difference in terms of digestion. So if you are in the habit of avoiding salt and you have no medical reason to do so, reconsider that. See what happens if you salt food to taste. The type of salt doesn't matter. True, some salts are refined and some have flow agents added to them, so if you want to be a purist, that is fine. You can use pure, unrefined sea salt or triple-blessed, high-mineral, super salt from pristine ancient sea beds somewhere in remote Canada or Siberia or whatever. And those unrefined salts *may* have some advantages over refined salt. But don't turn into a salt snob. Just eat some salt.

There's one more thing about salt that I'd like to mention. For people who have been restricting salt unnecessarily, sometimes liberal amounts of salt are useful in the beginning. Allow your taste to be your guide. If you find that you enjoy your food salty, then be generous with your use of salt. Over time, however, your desire for salt may wane. And, just as too little salt can lead to low stomach acid, too *much* salt can sometimes lead to high stomach acid levels. You'll know when you're eating too much salt because you might get some acid reflux, particularly when lying down. That happened to me after a while. I found that the same amount of salt that once had been therapeutic and delicious began to be slightly disagreeable. So I simply reduced the amount of salt I ate from obscene to moderate and the mild reflux went away. So be willing to adjust your salt intake up or down to find the sweet, er, I mean, salty spot.

Anti-Inflammatory

A lot of dietary advice these days proposes to reduce inflammation in the body by way of diet. Chronic inflammation is now being implicated as a possible cause of many conditions, including heart disease, diabetes, and cancer. The idea is that by reducing inflammation through diet, it is possible to reduce the risk of various diseases. As such, many people seek to follow the advice, believing that it will help them to be healthier. And, in fact, there *is* reason to believe that many digestive complaints may be helped by a reduction in inflammation.

The trouble comes from the fact that many of the anti-inflammatory diets (and there are many) are not actually anti-inflammatory; they're just *restrictive*. And, in fact, some of the foods that they may emphasize may actually be inflammatory while some of the foods that are restricted may be anti-inflammatory or at least *neutral*. And because many of the diets, when followed strictly, are likely to reduce caloric intake, the result may be *increased* inflammation due to insufficient calories and, therefore, increased stress.

Many so-called anti-inflammatory diets suggest that one should eliminate all refined grains. Why they suggest such a thing is unclear because I know of no studies demonstrating that refined grains are any more inflammatory than *unrefined* grains. And yet, most of the diets suggest that it is advisable to substitute whole grains in place of refined grains. The irony is that, as we've already seen, the bran in whole grains is irritating and thus *pro*-inflammatory whereas refined grain is neutral in that regard.

Some grain contains substances that some people cannot digest well. For example, a protein called gluten (actually a protein called gliadin contained in gluten) can cause an autoimmune (inflammatory) response in some people. For those who are sensitive to these substances, it may be best to avoid gluten grains altogether, but substituting *whole* grains for refined grains doesn't reduce inflammation in those cases; it merely adds yet more irritating substances. Eliminating gluten is *only* valuable for those people (estimated to be between 1 and 3 percent of the population) who are genuinely sensitive. Otherwise, eliminating categories of food is generally counterproductive.

Many anti-inflammatory diets suggest that one should eliminate all red meat and pork from one's diet. This suggestion is baseless, however. Yes, it is true that complete protein can be inflammatory. That is because some *essential* amino acids are inflammatory. However, this is *always* true, regardless of the source of the amino acids. And because they are *essential*, your body requires them. So whether you get them from fish or from beans or from beef, they will be equally inflammatory.

As we've already seen, sufficient *complete* protein is essential for digestive health. So cutting out red meat and pork because someone suggests that they are inflammatory is counterproductive. One researcher who has recently contributed to the notion that some animal foods are inflammatory and therefore unhealthy is a man named Colin T Campbell, the author of *The China Study*. However, what Campbell doesn't reveal in his book is that *according to his own experiments*, vegetable protein sources, which are supposedly anti-inflammatory, become equally inflammatory as soon as complementary amino acids are added to the diet. In other words, a dish of rice and beans is as inflammatory as beef.

What is rarely shared is that the inflammatory nature of complete protein can be completely offset by including adequate amounts of anti-inflammatory amino acids. Of particular note is the amino acid called glycine. Glycine is one of the most abundant amino acids in mammals as it is one of the major components of the most abundant type of protein in mammals--collagen. One of the easiest ways to include adequate glycine in the diet is to eat gelatin, which is collagen. You can find pork or beef gelatin in many grocery stores (unflavored Jello or Knox) or you can order specialty gelatin (Great Lakes is a popular brand among health food enthusiasts) on the internet.

Finally, many anti-inflammatory diets recommend reducing saturated fats. The trouble is that saturated fats occur in substantial amounts in many natural and healthy foods, including butter, beef, and coconut. Reducing saturated fat means reducing the intake of these foods that can contribute to health.

While it does seem to be true that saturated fats can be inflammatory, it's misleading to suggest that they are *always only* inflammatory. As it turns out, the experiments showing that saturated fats can be inflammatory also show that when sufficient omega-3 (polyunsaturated) fatty acids are included in the diet, the inflammatory effects disappear. Omega-6 polyunsaturated fat--the stuff found in large amounts in most "vegetable" oils such as soy, corn, and canola--is also inflammatory. However, unlike saturated fat, the studies show that nothing can offset the inflammation. In other words, if you eat a diet of real foods, including things like butter, lard, or fatty cuts of beef, which are composed of saturated, monounsaturated, and polyunsaturated fats (both small amounts of omega-6 and omega-3), then the total effect will *not* be inflammatory. In fact, many of those natural fats also contain anti-inflammatory compounds such as butyric acid that offer a lot of health benefits. Plus, you'll get the benefit of sufficient fat-soluble vitamins, cholesterol, protein, and lots of other vitamins (choline, B vitamins, and so forth) that are found in many of these healthy foods.

A truly anti-inflammatory diet can be helpful in the quest to improve digestion. And a truly anti-inflammatory diet is one that first and foremost includes enough calories. It should also include sufficient fat, protein, and carbohydrates while minimizing irritating forms of fiber. If one is sensitive to gluten, then eliminating gluten can be anti-inflammatory, but for everyone else eliminating gluten will not be beneficial. And supplementing with gelatin can help to make sure that the protein intake will be balanced by anti-inflammatory amino acids. Add to that some fresh fruit and you've got the makings of an anti-inflammatory diet that can actually work. The key is that it is largely *inclusive* rather than restrictive.

Fasting

Yet another way in which many people worsen their digestive health is through extended fasting. Each of us already typically fasts for 8 to 10 hours or more every night. While *healthy* people may experience benefits (or at least no harm) in fasting for as long as 24 or even 48 hours on occasion, people with impaired digestion will generally not experience benefits from fasting.

One of the ways in which fasting is often promoted to those with digestive problems is by claiming that fasting "gives the digestive system a rest." This conjures up an image of a much overworked stomach and intestines catching some needed Zs in a hammock on some tropical island. Yet while it *sounds* nice, it's just not true.

Again, there are differences between truly healthy people and those who are not. A healthy person will suffer no harm from fasting for a day. Her or his metabolism will remain healthy, and she or he is fully capable of burning stored fuel (i.e. fat) for energy without excessive stress for short periods of time.

However, for anyone with an impaired metabolic rate or digestive system, fasting for more than the typical evening fast is counterproductive.

While fasting, the body will use stored glycogen to fuel the brain and muscles. Once glycogen stores become depleted, the body will next start using either adipose tissue or muscle tissue or some combination of the two. In most people, this necessitates the production of large amounts of stress hormones.

For most people, eating regularly will be the best way to improve digestion. Many people with poor digestion are in the habit of eating only once or twice a day. Yet for most people, it will be best to eat *at least* three times a day. And in the beginning, it may be best to eat more often, even six or more time per day if necessary in order to eat enough calories.

Some people with poor digestion find it uncomfortable to eat three times a day because they still feel full long after they eat a meal. In that case, it is important to eat *more often*. The way to achieve that is to eat less in a meal and focus on easily digested foods. By eating small amounts of them often, you can begin to increase your metabolic rate, making it easier to eat more food.

Over time, you will likely find that you can eat larger meals less frequently while maintaining a healthy digestive system and metabolic rate. However, that may take time. When in doubt, eat smaller meals more often and/or snack often. Your goal is to avoid fasting for long periods of time and to make sure that you eat *at least* three times every day. Obviously you needn't become obsessive about that, but neither should you continue with the status quo of skipping breakfast and/or lunch every day if that's not working well for you. Make a concerted effort to eat more frequently in that case.

Laxatives

Many people who have digestive problems have tried laxatives at least once. Laxatives are of many types, including herbs like senna or cascara sagrada (often marketed as "cleanses"), drugs like polyethylene glycol (Miralax), and poorly absorbed forms of the mineral magnesium.

Although laxatives can offer some temporary sense of relief from bloating or feelings of constipation that can sometimes accompany digestive problems, in the long run they are not a good idea. Many laxatives can become habit-forming, and they generally disturb electrolyte balance and normal function of the digestive system.

Constipation and bloating often accompany poor digestion that is caused by low BMR. If you experience these symptoms, then laxatives won't fix the cause. Instead, you need to eat more and rest more.

Candida

Candida albicans is a yeast organism that lives in and on most of us all of the time. And for most people most of the time, it is not a problem at all. Sometimes, however, candida can flourish and the result is what is called an overgrowth. The most common candida overgrowth types are vaginal yeast infections and thrush (overgrowth in the mouth and throat). Candida *can* spread to other places in the body and problems can result. It *is* possible to have systemic candida overgrowth, meaning that candida can multiply in the blood. And candida may spread to the small intestine and stomach. However, I suspect that this happens both more often than conventional doctors usually like to believe and far *less* often than most alternative health practitioners like to believe.

In any case, many people are absolutely convinced that they are suffering from the dreaded candida, by which what they surely *really* mean is candida overgrowth of some sort. Normally, since the complaints are of a digestive sort (bloating, etc.), we can assume that the candida overgrowth, real or imaginary, is happening (or not) in the digestive system, meaning mostly in the small intestine and stomach.

Unfortunately, the most common advice for how to remedy candida overgrowth is to "starve" it by avoiding all sugar, which usually involves not only eliminating white and brown sugar, maple syrup, and honey, but also all fruit and starch and even most dairy. In other words, many "anti-candida" diets are low-carbohydrate diets. Not only is this advice unproven, but it actually is likely to worsen some of the factors that may actually contribute to candida overgrowth in the first place.

Low carbohydrate diets are often (though not always) necessarily low-calorie diets. Remember, your goal is to eat 3500-4000 calories *minimum* per day in order to restore digestive health. Try doing that while eating only meat and butter. If you're like most people, you'll feel nauseous before you can do it. And since low calorie means low metabolic rate and low metabolic rate means *reduced immunity* and *slower digestion* plus *leaky gut*, you're setting yourself up for worsening symptoms.

Let's suppose for a moment that candida really does need sugar to survive and that it is possible to starve it by eliminating all sugar and starch. A critical evaluation quickly reveals that this strategy will never work *unless* you are willing to die first. That's because like candida, your body needs sugar. In fact, your body needs sugar so much that even if you eat no carbohydrates at all, your body will *produce* sugar in order to feed your brain. Without sugar even for a minute, your brain will die. So let's say that you eliminate all carbohydrates from your diet. Your body will produce sugar to feed your brain, and guess what? That darn candida will eat it too and stay alive.

Finally, as we've already seen, candida is not the only organism that needs carbohydrates to survive; the 90 percent of your body that isn't human depends upon them, too. And you depend upon those organisms. So if you eliminate all carbohydrates in an attempt to starve candida, you'll not only fail, but you'll likely starve your body, both the human cells and the non-human cells alike.

So if you are concerned about candida overgrowth, then my advice, which is contrary to most of what you'll find on the internet and elsewhere, is as follows. First of all, eat enough, including carbohydrates. You need lots of calories to fuel a healthy metabolic rate. You need lots of carbohydrates to feed the healthy bacteria in your body. In addition, you should sleep a lot, rest a lot, and learn to relax.

Sleep

Most of this book has been about food. That's because the food part is the most complicated to communicate. But that doesn't mean that it's the most important. *Just as important* are getting enough quality sleep and learning how to relax. Although these subjects are much easier to write about in a shorter space, don't underestimate their importance.

Sleep is a vitally important subject that often goes overlooked. Numerous studies now show that adults generally require *at least* 7 hours of quality sleep every single night, and many adults require 8 or 9 hours of sleep every night.

Although correlation doesn't prove causation, it is worth noting that a number of epidemiological studies show that less than 7 or 8 hours of sleep per night is strongly correlated with all kinds of health problems, including cardiovascular disease, diabetes, and cancer. I don't know of any studies that specifically look at whether digestive problems correlate with a lack of sleep, but you can bet there is one.

Insufficient sleep is shown to increase adrenaline, alter cortisol patterns, and alter T3 levels. Chronic lack of sleep can alter metabolic rate. So if you're not sleeping enough, consider the importance that adequate sleep can have in regard to your general health and your digestive health.

Many people with poor digestion complain that they wake early in the morning, unable to get back to sleep. They often say that they wake to racing thoughts or a sense of urgency or even panic. If you experience this, it is a very good indication that you are not eating enough. Often, eating more will help to resolve this. Meanwhile, if you wake in the early morning, then eat some quickly-digested sugar and a pinch of salt. That may help you to get back to sleep.

If the quality of your sleep is poor, that will also have negative impacts on your health and digestion. If you know that you snore or breathe through your mouth at night, then that can adversely affect the quality of your sleep. Many people find that correcting these issues can help tremendously. Although crude, some people find that lightly taping the mouth shut with medical tape can help train one to breathe through the nose at night. A word of caution, however. Should you choose to do that, ensure that the tape is snug enough to gently remind the mouth to stay shut, but don't attempt to use tape to force the mouth to stay shut as it is a good idea to continue to allow for the possibility to breathe through the mouth should the genuine need arise.

Relax

Learning how to relax is an extremely important and valuable skill that can greatly contribute to digestive health. This is a skill that is often overlooked, and yet it can be one of the most useful, not only for improving digestion, but also for improving the quality of life more generally.

To begin with, let's look at the most obvious (and yet often overlooked) ways in which relaxing can help with digestion. In today's culture with a tremendous emphasis on appearance and being thin, many of us suck in our belly without even realizing it. Furthermore, tension in the abdomen is often a way in which we habitually seek to "protect" ourselves from everything from money worries to being late for an appointment.

All the tension that many of us hold in our abdomens can have seriously negative impacts on our digestive health in a number of ways. First of all, simply holding all that tension physically restricts the amount of space available for holding and moving food. So by learning to relax the belly, more space literally gets opened up.

Secondly, tension in the abdomen interferes with natural, normal breathing, which relies on the free movement of the thoracic diaphragm. Not only does that interfere with breathing, but it impairs digestion as well as immune function. Normally, the slow, rhythmic up and down movement of the thoracic diaphragm massages the organs of the abdomen. However, when the belly is held in chronic tension, that massaging action doesn't occur.

Learning to free your belly can be a hugely liberating experience, and it is one that I highly recommend. But it requires being willing to allow of some of the fears and anxieties that chronic belly tension seeks to control. The good news is that it's never as bad as we fear it will be.

To relax your belly, the main thing you can do is allow it to hang out. Even the skinniest of us (I was one of the super skinny at my worst with a dangerously low weight and feeling unable to eat) can let our belly hang out. From the bottom of the ribcage all the way to the groin, release the muscular contraction that habitually sucks in the belly. You may find that it helps to place your hands on your belly and feel your belly gently filling and resting in your hands. Gently rub and shake your belly to release any tension. Allow it to be totally relaxed.

Although tension in the belly is the most obvious way in which tension is associated with digestive problems, all other tension is also linked to digestive problems. The reason is that chronic tension anywhere in the body is a sign of stress of some kind. Whether the stress has an emotional component or it is purely physiological (i.e. a habit of physical tension), the effects are more or less the same. And some of the effects include slowing down the digestive process, reducing stomach acid, and other things that may be useful if you're trying to outrun a hungry tiger but not so helpful if you're trying to eat.

Most of us distinguish between emotional stress and purely physiological stress. However, that isn't generally useful. When it comes to *all* types of stress, what I have found is that the most effective manner in which to release the stress (and thereby improve digestion), whether it's a stiff neck or a chronic sense of anxiety, is to soften and relax the physical tension in the body. My best and simplest recommendation in this regard is to simply scan the body any time there is any sense of stress, worry, anxiety, fear, or physical discomfort and notice where there is tension. Then, simply allow for the tension to relax to whatever degree possible. Repeat the process as many times as necessary.

The process that I just described is ridiculously simple, yet it is extremely powerful. Of course it is not the *only* way to release stress. There are lots of techniques available. But that is by far the most effective I have ever come across, and it can help digestion tremendously, particularly when done during and following eating so as to relax a lot of the low level tension and anxiety that many of us hold without even being aware of it.

It's also worth mentioning that eating more tends to lead to relaxation. So even though it can be challenging at first, the more you eat (and the more you consciously relax), the easier it is to eat and relax. This is what I call a "kind cycle" versus a vicious cycle, and you'll notice that it mirrors the vicious cycle that happens from eating less and stressing more. So when it doubt, relax and eat, eat and relax.

Weight Gain

For some people who have digestive problems, gaining weight is a godsend. Yet for others, weight gain is unwelcomed. The truth is that in order to repair poor digestion, most people will gain weight initially. If you see that as a good sign, then that is wonderful. If you don't want to gain weight, then the weight gain can be a trigger for stress.

I'd like to remind you of the earlier discussion about set point theory. Remember that the starving Minnesotans ate *massive* amounts of food for 9 months in order to restore their metabolisms and their weights. In doing so they initially overshot their starting weights by 10 percent. They only restored their original, lower weights by continuing to eat lots of food.

You'll also recall that despite the fact that the Vermonters were eating 10,000 calories a day with the goal of gaining 25 percent of their starting weights, they couldn't reach their target weight. They gained weight, but eventually stalled out, and with their greatly increased metabolic rates, as soon as they stopped eating massive amounts of food and returned to normal eating, the weight fell off.

According to set point theory, you can only lose or gain weight within a limited range before your metabolism will adjust. The set point can move up or down based on various lifestyle and environmental factors. Ironically, the less you eat, the *higher* your set point gets whereas the more that you eat, the lower the set point. What that means is that after undereating for a while, your set point will raise so that when you begin to eat enough you will gain weight above your previous set point. However, once you continue to eat enough, your set point will lower and you will effortlessly lose weight while still eating the same amount of food.

This advice runs counter to much of what weight loss companies want you to think. But there is good evidence that it is so. What this means is that you may gain weight while restoring your metabolic and digestive health. But if you continue to eat enough, sleep enough, and relax enough, your set point will likely settle at a weight that feels good for you.

Summary

For those of us who have experienced digestive hell, we know how challenging and hopeless it can feel. When even the "safe" foods stop working, that can be a scary time. Out of desperation, we may turn to one extreme recommendation to another--fasting, cleansing, restrictive diets, and so on--but nothing seems to work.

My message for you in this book is that for many of us it is possible to improve digestion by eating more, sleeping more, and relaxing more. By making these things a priority, it is possible heal your metabolism, reduce stress and inflammation, and start to feel better.

Eating more when digestion is already poor can seem like an impossibility. However, it is generally possible with some flexibility, willingness, and creativity. When I first began to heal, I ate a *lot* of milk, sugar, cheese, butter, and potatoes along with smaller amounts of other foods because that is what worked for me. Of course, you may be different. What works best for you may be Twinkies and hamburgers or pizza or maybe you're one of the bone broth and Ho Hos sorts. What is required is to focus on highly palatable, energy-dense foods that work *for you* and find an eating pattern that works for you. For example, many people will find that emphasizing easy-to-digest sugars, fats, and protein sources will be easier than trying to eat lots of whole grains and kale. And many people find initially that it may be easier to eat smaller, more frequent meals than to try to eat infrequent, large meals. In any case, be willing to experiment and find what works best for you. And be willing to keep experimenting and adapting to the changing needs of your body as you heal. Listen to your body's tastes and desires. They will serve as good guides along the way. When you desire certain foods, be willing to eat them.

A lot of people who find themselves in digestive hell have a history of eating "healthy" foods. And for many, letting go of the ideas of what is healthy and what is unhealthy can be a major challenge and a major obstacle to healing. That's because what is healthy in the context of healing the digestive system when the metabolic rate is low and when stress is high is *energy-dense* and *palatable*. That is often the opposite of what we normally think of as health food--things like celery and wheatgrass juice or brown rice and kale.

If you struggle with letting go of the ideologically-based ideas about what you should or shouldn't eat, then consider this: at least for most of us there was a time in our childhood when we ate with reckless abandon. We didn't worry about whether it was GMO or whole grain or how much vitamin C it contained. We didn't care about anything except whether we were hungry and it tasted good. That was it. Or maybe that wasn't you. Maybe you were one of those kids who had digestive problems. But you can at least see that lots of other people with good digestion are able to eat *just about anything*.

We all have preferences, some of them ideological. That is fine. Personally, I prefer fresh, local, organic, preferably raised by me when it comes to food. I prefer real food, not industrially produced stuff. And I suspect that it not only tastes better to me, but it's probably healthier. But when it comes to healing, the mistake that many people make is that they insist on ideological purity while sacrificing energy-density and palatability. Sure, the locally-grown romaine lettuce and heirloom tomato may be more "pure" than, say, a Twinkie or a pizza from some chain restaurant. But you just can't eat enough of the lettuce and tomato to satisfy your body's energy needs. I am not suggesting that it is impossible to maintain ideological purity while also eating enough calories, but I am suggesting that at the very least you must prioritize energy (calorie) needs before ideology. And in that context, as offensive as it may be to many of our sensibilities, our "pure" and holy "health" foods are often the worst things we could be eating, at least for now. I mean, if you want to sneak in some kale for dessert after you've finished off 4500 calories for the day, then that is fine. But for the love of your metabolism, don't begin breakfast with a green smoothie.

Eating enough is essential, but that is not the only thing that is important. You'll also want to make sure that you are getting adequate *quality* sleep *every* night (or at least as often as possible). And learning to relax the body in *all* situations can greatly reduce stress and improve hormonal balance, which will have positive effects on digestive health.

Give the suggestions in this book a sincere try and see what happens. Of course, in the current social context in which we're being told to eat less, hit the gym several times a day, sleep less, and do more, the suggestions in this book may seem radical. But if ever you are in doubt, keep in mind that all I'm suggesting is what has been common sense for most of human history; eat enough, sleep enough, relax. That's all. I'm definitely *not* suggesting that you do anything extreme. Please understand that when I suggest minimum calorie targets of 3500-4000 calories, I am not offering that as a *rule*. It's just a guideline that may be useful as a goal. The point of which is to ask you to challenge yourself to eat enough. For many people, 3500-4000 calories a day really will be the minimum necessary in order to heal, but always respect your body and your present needs. Challenge yourself, but also listen to your body and be gentle and kind. Please don't turn my suggestions into yet another heroic, macho attempt to force anything. Then they are no better than the typical suggestions to restrict, fast, and otherwise push yourself to extremes.

I wish you the best in your recovery of digestive health. May you eat well, rest well, and live well.

Get My Future Books FREE

If you enjoyed this book (Hey, if you made it this far it couldn't have been that bad), you'll probably enjoy many of my other books about health and wellness. And you can get all my new releases in health and wellness for free by signing up for my mailing list at www.joeylotthealth.com. It's simple, it's free, and it's totally honest and legitimate. Nothing scammy or spammy or anything else like that (i.e. I won't be trying to sell you The 7 Dirty Underground Top Secret Weird Tricks for Rock Hard Abs or Young Living Oils). It's just about free books for those who appreciate my work, because I appreciate YOU. Simple as that.

Connect with Me

I welcome your questions, comments, and feedback of any kind. Please feel free to email me at joeylott@gmail.com. I am now receiving so many emails that I cannot always reply to every email. I do read them all, and I do my best to reply to as many as possible. For the benefit of others, I may choose to publish my response to your email on my blog or in book format. I will maintain your privacy and anonymity if I choose to publish my response.

One Small Favor

My sincere goal in writing is to share something that may be of value to you. And I endeavor to do so while keeping the costs low for readers. The success of my books and my ability to reach other readers who may benefit from my books depends in large part on having lots of thoughtful, honest reviews written about my work. You would do me a great favor if you would please take a moment to generously write a review of this book at Amazon.com. This will only take a few minutes of your time, and you will be helping me a great deal. I sure would appreciate it.

Free Video Series

I also have a site at www.peacefulpossibility.com where I have over three hours of free video training on a handful of limbic system retraining techniques, including the Big Chill. On that site I share more detailed instruction. Everything on the site is completely free. Nothing is for sale there.

About the Author

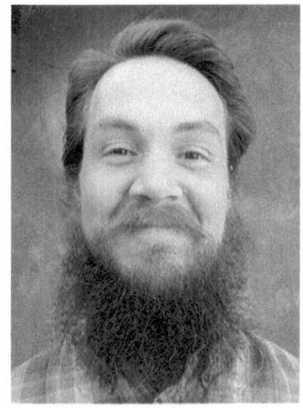

"The secret to happiness is to let go of everything - see through every assumption."

Beginning at a young age Joey Lott experienced intensifying anxiety. For several decades he lived with restrictive eating disorders, obsessions, compulsions, and an inescapable fear. By the time he was 30 years old he was physically sick, emotionally volatile, and mentally obsessed with keeping any and all unwanted thoughts and experiences at bay.

At this time Lott was living on a futon mattress in a tiny cabin in the woods. He was so sick that he could barely move. He was deeply depressed and hopeless. All this despite doing all the "right" things such as years of meditation, yoga, various "perfect" diets, clean air, and pure water.

Just when things were at their most dire, a crack appeared in the conceptual world that had formerly been mistaken for reality. By peering into this crack and underneath all the assumptions that had been unquestioned up to that moment, Lott began a great undoing. The revelation of this undoing is that reality is utterly simple, ever-present, seamless, and indivisible.

Lott's books provide a glimpse into the seamless, simple, and joyous nature of reality, offering a glimpse through the crack in conceptual worlds. Whether writing about the ultimate non-dual nature of reality, eating disorders, stress, disease, or any other subject, he offers the invitation to look at things differently, leaving behind the old, out-grown, painful limitations we have used to bind ourselves in suffering. And then, he welcomes you home to the effortless simplicity of yourself as you are.

Not sure where to begin? Pick up a copy of Lott's most popular book, *You're Trying Too Hard*, which strips away all the concepts that keep us searching for a greater, more spiritual, more peaceful life or self.